MEDITERRANEAN DIET BREKFAST RECIPES

LEARN HOW TO COOK MEDITERRANEAN THROUGH THIS DETAILED COOKBOOK, COMPLETE OF SEVERAL TASTY IDEAS FOR A GOOD AND HEALTY BREAKFAST. SUITABLE FOT BOYTH ADULTS AND KIDS, IT WILL HELP YOU LOSE WEIGHT AND FEEL BETTER, WITHOUT GIVING UP YOUR FAVOURITE FOOD

Table of contents

Berries Porridge 8

Olives and Greens Salad 9

Lime Kale Bowls 10

Spinach Almond Smoothie 11

Banana Bowls 12

Pear and Nuts Oatmeal 13

Apple Coconut Oats 14

Fruit and Chia Bowls 15

Red Smoothie 16

Egg Bowls 17

Cherries Bowls 18

Ginger Smoothie 19

Chia Porridge 20

Mint Cucumber Salad 21

Quinoa Bowls 22

Smoothie Bowls 23

Grape and Oats Bowls 24

Rhubarb Bowls 25

Kale Smoothie 26

Vanilla Quinoa Mix 27

Spinach and Eggs Mix 28

Pancakes 29

Veggie Muffins 30

Almond Green Eggs 31

Honey Apple Bowls 32

Peppers and Olives Bowls 33

Chives Sweet Potato Mix 34

Avocado and Spinach Salad 35

Turmeric Eggs and Sprouts 36

Lime Spinach Bowls 37

Spinach and Collard Greens Bowls 38

Quinoa and Eggs Bowls 39

Barley and Kale Salad 40
Sweet Potato and Carrots Mix 41
Cucumber and Basil Mix 42
Zucchinis and Arugula Bowls..43
Eggs and Scallions Mix...44
Almond Frittata 45
Blueberries Bowls 46
Balsamic Spinach Salad..47
Parsley Potato Bowls 48
Parsley Eggs...49
Coconut Maple Oatmeal..50
Coconut Broccoli Mix 51
Green Olives Bowls 52
Tomato and Spring Onions Salad 53
Citrus Pear Salad 54
Cantaloupe Bowls 55
Cauliflower and Eggs Pan...56
Berries and Walnuts Oats 57
Spinach and Avocado Smoothie..58
Arugula, Beets and Tomato Salad 59
Quinoa Bowls...60
Carrots and Quinoa Mix 61
Tomato and Scallions Salad 62
Black Beans Mix...63
Onion, Corn and Avocado Salad 64
Basil Eggs..65
Zucchini Spread 66
Watermelon Salad 67
Mango Coconut Oatmeal...68
Cherries Oats...69
Pecan Oats 70
Creamy Peaches...71
Maple Yogurt Bowls..72
Pomegranate Oatmeal 73
Chia Bowls..74
Carrots Hash...75

Peppers and Eggs Mix....................76
Parsley Eggs....................77
Artichoke Eggs Mix....................78
Beans and Eggs....................79
Mozzarella Scramble....................80
Cheddar Hash Browns....................81
Chives Rice Mix....................82
Cinnamon Quinoa....................83
Cherries Mix....................84
Plum and Sunflower Mix....................85
Apples and Cinnamon Yogurt....................86
Almond Strawberry Bowls....................87
Almond Peach Mix....................88
Almond Rice....................89
Figs Yogurt....................90
Coconut Porridge....................91
Brown Rice Mix....................92
Vanilla Rice....................93
Cherries Rice....................94
Ginger and Almond Rice....................95
Minced Hash Mix....................96
Mushroom and Cheddar Mix....................97
Tomato Eggs....................98
Paprika Omelet....................99
Cinnamon Zucchini and Oats....................100
Maple Almonds Bowl....................101
Chickpeas and Cucumber Salad....................102
Millet Mix....................103
Ginger Chia Pudding....................104
Cinnamon Tapioca Bowls....................105
Coconut Hash....................106
Snow Peas and Scallions Bowls....................107
Coconut Chickpeas Mix....................108
Lime Peppers Salad....................109
Green Beans Mix....................110
Eggs Salad....................111

Vanilla Berries 112

Apples and Blueberries Mix 113

Buckwheat Bowls 114

Cauliflower Salad 115

Chicken and Pepper Mix 116

Beef Bowl 117

Smoked Salmon and Eggs Mix 118

Cheesy Asparagus Mix 119

Stuffed Avocados 120

Eggs with Spinach and Chicken 121

Ham and Mushroom Scramble 122

Spinach and Chicken Frittata 123

Boiled Eggs 124

Shrimp and Mushroom Mix 125

Chorizo and Pork Mix 126

Sausage and Spinach Mix 127

7

Berries Porridge

Prep time: 10 minutes **ICooking time:** 20 minutes ı **Servings:** 4

Ingredients:
- 2 cups almond milk
- ½ cup almonds, chopped
- 1 pear, peeled and cubed
- ½ cup blueberries
- 1 teaspoon ginger, grated
- 1 teaspoon maple syrup

Directions:
1. In a pot, combine the almond milk with the almonds and the other ingredients, toss, bring to a simmer and cook over medium heat for 20 minutes.
2. Divide into bowls and serve.

Nutrition facts per serving: calories 381, fat 34.7, fiber 5.7, carbs 18.6, protein 5.6

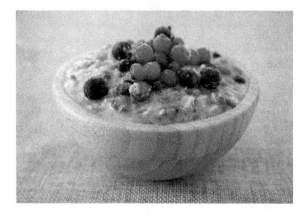

Olives and Greens Salad

Prep time: 5 minutes I **Cooking time:** 0 minutes I **Servings:** 2

Ingredients:
- 2 cups baby spinach
- 1 tablespoon avocado oil
- 1 cup blueberries
- ½ cup black olives, pitted and halved
- 1 avocado, peeled, pitted and halved

Directions:
1. In a bowl, combine the spinach with the berries and the other ingredients, toss, divide into smaller bowls and serve for breakfast.

Nutrition facts per serving: calories 301, fat 24.5, fiber 10.5, carbs 22.7, protein 3.7

Lime Kale Bowls

Prep time: 5 minutes **I Cooking time:** 0 minutes **I Servings:** 4

Ingredients:
- 1 pound baby kale
- 1 cup kalamata olives, pitted and halved
- ½ cup green olives, pitted and halved
- 2 tablespoons olive oil
- 2 tablespoons apple cider vinegar
- Juice of 1 lime
- A pinch of white pepper

Directions:
1. In a salad bowl, combine the kale with the olives and the other ingredients, toss, divide into smaller bowls and serve.

Nutrition facts per serving: calories 165, fat 11.4, fiber 3.9, carbs 15.2, protein 4.3

Spinach Almond Smoothie

Prep time: 5 minutes ı **Cooking time:** 0 minutes I **Servings:** 2

Ingredients:
- 1 cup baby spinach
- 1 avocado, peeled, pitted and mashed
- ½ cup almond milk
- ¼ cup water
- 1 cup raspberries
- 1 banana, peeled and sliced

Directions:
1. In a blender, combine the spinach with the avocado, and the other ingredients, pulse well, divide into 2 glasses and serve for breakfast.

Nutrition facts per serving: calories 431, fat 34.6, fiber 13.9, carbs 33.3, protein 5.1

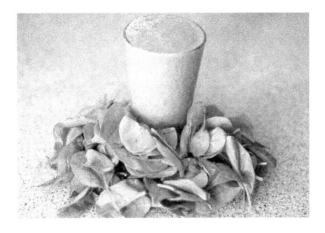

Banana Bowls

Prep time: 5 minutes I **Cooking time:** 5 minutes I **Servings:** 6

Ingredients:
- 2 cups coconut milk
- ½ cup coconut, unsweetened and shredded
- ¼ teaspoon ginger, ground
- 2 bananas, peeled and sliced
- ¼ teaspoon cinnamon powder

Directions:
1. Heat up the milk in a small pot over medium heat, add the coconut and the other ingredients, cook for 5 minutes, toss gently, divide into bowls and serve.

Nutrition facts per serving: calories 243, fat 21.4, fiber 3.4, carbs 14.5, protein 2.5

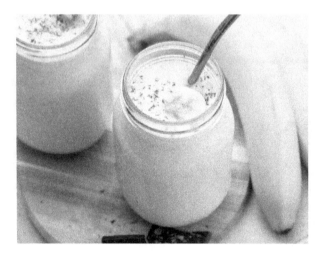

Pear and Nuts Oatmeal

Prep time: 15 minutes I **Cooking time:** 0 minutes I **Servings:** 2

Ingredients:
- 1 cup old-fashioned oats
- ½ cup almond milk
- 1 tablespoon maple syrup
- 2 pears, peeled and cubed
- 1 tablespoon walnuts, chopped
- 1 tablespoon almonds, blanched and chopped

Directions:
1. In a bowl, combine the oats with the milk and the other ingredients, toss, leave aside for 15 minutes, divide into smaller bowls and serve.

Nutrition facts per serving: calories 476, fat 21, fiber 12.4, carbs 69.9, protein 9

Apple Coconut Oats

Prep time: 5 minutes I **Cooking time:** 10 minutes I **Servings:** 2

Ingredients:
- 1 cup coconut milk
- ½ cup old-fashioned oats
- 1 apple, cored and cubed
- 1 teaspoon turmeric powder
- 2 teaspoons maple syrup

Directions:
1. Put the milk in a pan, heat it up over medium heat, add the oats and the other ingredients, toss, simmer for 10 minutes, divide into bowls and serve.

Nutrition facts per serving: calories 430, fat 30.4, fiber 7.6, carbs 40.7, protein 5.6

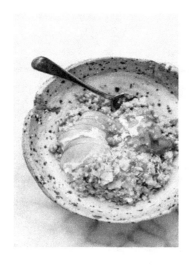

Fruit and Chia Bowls

Prep time: 5 minutes I **Cooking time:** 0 minutes I **Servings:** 2

Ingredients:
- 1 cup pineapple, peeled and cubed
- 1 banana, peeled
- 1 apple, core d and cubed
- 1 teaspoon chia seeds
- 1 tablespoon lime juice
- ½ tablespoon avocado oil

Directions:
1. In a bowl, combine the pineapple with the banana and the other ingredients, toss, divide into smaller bowls and serve for breakfast,

Nutrition facts per serving: calories 225, fat 5.3, fiber 10.4, carbs 45.9, protein 3.8

Red Smoothie

Prep time: 5 minutes I **Cooking time:** 0 minutes I **Servings:** 2

Ingredients:
- 2 cups almond milk
- 1 cup cherries, pitted
- ½ banana, peeled and frozen
- 1 tablespoon coconut butter

Directions:
1. In your blender, combine the milk with the cherries and the other ingredients, pulse well, divide into glasses and serve.

Nutrition facts pers serving: calories 678, fat 81.3, fiber 6.6, carbs 35.5, protein 7.3

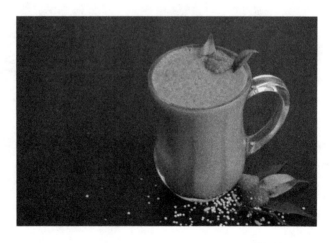

Egg Bowls

Prep time: 5 minutes I **Cooking time:** 15 minutes I **Servings:** 4

Ingredients:
- 2 tablespoons olive oil
- 1 yellow onion, chopped
- 8 eggs, whisked
- A pinch of salt and black pepper
- 1 teaspoon coriander, ground
- 1 tablespoon chives, chopped
- 1 tablespoon rosemary, chopped
- 1 tablespoon cilantro, chopped
- 1 tablespoon parsley, chopped

Directions:
1. Heat up a pan with the oil over medium heat, add the onion, stir and sauté for 3 minutes.
2. Add the eggs and the other ingredients, toss, cook for 12 minutes more, divide into bowls and serve for breakfast.

Nutrition facts per serving: calories 200, fat 15.9, fiber 1, carbs 3.9, protein 11.5

Cherries Bowls

Prep time: 5 minutes I **Cooking time:** 0 minutes I **Servings:** 4

Ingredients:
- 1 cup almond milk
- 1 cup pears, cored and cubed
- 1 cup cherries, pitted and halved
- ½ teaspoon vanilla extract
- 1 tablespoon cocoa powder
- 2 tablespoons walnuts, chopped

Directions:
1. In a bowl, mix the pears with the cherries and the other ingredients, toss, divide into smaller bowls and serve for breakfast.

Nutrition facts per serving: calories 211, fat 16.9, fiber 3.4, carbs 15.8, protein 2.8

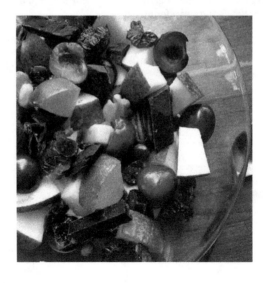

Ginger Smoothie

Prep time: 5 minutes I **Cooking time:** 0 minutes I **Servings:** 2

Ingredients:
- 1 cup almond milk
- 2 mangoes, peeled and cubed
- 1 tablespoon ginger, grated
- ½ cup water
- 1 teaspoon nutmeg, ground
- 1 tablespoon maple syrup

Directions:
1. In your blender, combine the mangoes with the milk and the other ingredients, pulse well, divide into glasses and serve for breakfast.

Nutrition facts per serving: calories 519, fat 30.5, fiber 8.6, carbs 66.1, protein 5.8

Chia Porridge

Prep time: 5 minutes I **Cooking time:** 5 minutes I **Servings:** 4

Ingredients:
- 1 cup walnuts, chopped and toasted
- 3 tablespoons chia seeds
- 2 cups almond milk
- ¼ cup coconut, shredded and toasted
- 1 banana, peeled and mashed
- 1 tablespoon coconut oil, melted
- ½ teaspoon turmeric powder

Directions:
1. Heat up a pot with the milk over medium heat, add the chia seeds, the walnuts and the other ingredients, toss, simmer for 5 minutes, divide into bowls and serve warm for breakfast.

Nutrition facts per serving: calories 647, fat 58.8, fiber 13.4, carbs 26.4, protein 14.3

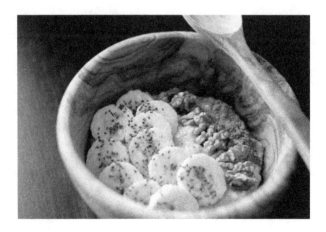

Mint Cucumber Salad

Prep time: 5 minutes I **Cooking time:** 0 minutes I **Servings:** 2

Ingredients:
- 1 cup mango, peeled and cubed
- 1 cup cucumber, peeled and cubed
- Juice of ½ lime
- 1 teaspoon ginger powder
- ¼ teaspoon turmeric powder
- 1 teaspoon mint, dried
- 1 tablespoon chia seeds
- 1 tablespoon chives, chopped

Directions:
1. In a bowl, combine the mango with the cucumber, the lime juice and the other ingredients, toss, divide into smaller bowls and serve for breakfast.

Nutrition facts per serving: calories 68, fat 0.5, fiber 2, carbs 17.1, protein 1.3

Quinoa Bowls

Prep time: 5 minutes I **Cooking time:** 0 minutes I **Servings:** 6

Ingredients:
- 1 cup cherries, pitted and halved
- 2 cups quinoa, cooked
- 1 banana, peeled and sliced
- 2 teaspoons maple syrup
- 1 tablespoon mint, chopped

Directions:
1. In a bowl, combine the quinoa with the cherries and the other ingredients, toss, divide into smaller bowls and serve for breakfast.

Nutrition facts per serving: calories 247, fat 3.5, fiber 4.6, carbs 45.9, protein 8.3

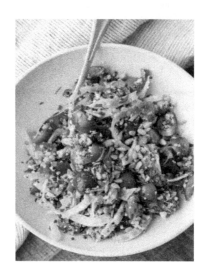

Smoothie Bowls

Prep time: 5 minutes I **Cooking time:** 0 minutes I **Servings:** 2

Ingredients:
- 1 avocado, pitted and peeled
- 1 cup coconut milk
- 1 cup water
- 1 banana, peeled and mashed
- 1 tablespoon lime juice
- 1 cup baby spinach

Directions:
1. In your blender, combine the avocados with the milk, the water and the remaining ingredients, pulse well, divide into bowls and serve.

Nutrition facts per serving: calories 125, fat 6, fiber 7, carbs 9, protein 4

Grape and Oats Bowls

Prep time: 5 minutes |**Cooking time:** 15 minutes | **Servings:** 4

Ingredients:
- 1 cup steel cut oats
- 2 cups almond milk
- ½ cup grapes, halved
- ½ teaspoon vanilla extract
- 1 and ½ tablespoons cinnamon powder
- ¼ teaspoon ginger, ground
- ¼ teaspoon cardamom, ground

Directions:
1. Heat up a pot with the milk over medium heat, add the oats, the grapes and the other ingredients, toss, cook for about 15 minutes, divide into bowls and serve.

Nutrition facts per serving: calories 188, fat 12.4, fiber 6, carbs 13, protein 6

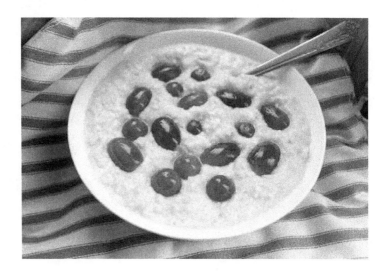

Rhubarb Bowls

Prep time: 10 minutes I **Cooking time:** 10 minutes I **Servings:** 4

Ingredients:
- ½ teaspoon ginger, grated
- ½ teaspoon cinnamon powder
- 1 cup rhubarb, sliced
- 1 cup cherries, pitted and halved
- 1 apple, cored, peeled and chopped
- 2 cups almond milk
- 1 teaspoon vanilla extract

Directions:
1. Heat up a pot with the milk over medium heat, add the rhubarb, the cherries and the other ingredients, toss, cook for 10 minutes, divide into bowls and serve cold for breakfast.

Nutrition facts per serving: calories 200, fat 6.5, fiber 6, carbs 13, protein 2.3

Kale Smoothie

Prep time: 5 minutes I **Cooking time:** 0 minutes I **Servings:** 4

Ingredients:
- 2 cups grapes, halved
- 2 cups almond milk
- 1 cup water
- 1 banana, frozen and peeled
- 1 cup baby kale
- 2 tablespoons maple syrup

Directions:
1. In blender, combine the grapes with the milk and the other ingredients, pulse well, divide into glasses and serve for breakfast.

Nutrition facts per serving: calories 125, fat 3, fiber 6, carbs 14, protein 8

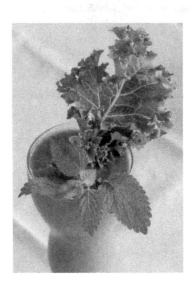

Vanilla Quinoa Mix

Prep time: 10 minutes I **Cooking time:** 0 minutes I **Servings:** 4

Ingredients:
- 2 cups quinoa, cooked
- 1 cup sunflower seeds
- 1 cup pumpkin seeds
- 1 cup almond milk
- 1 tablespoon coconut oil
- 1 teaspoon vanilla extract
- 1 teaspoon ginger, grated

Directions:
1. In a large bowl, combine the quinoa with the seeds and the other ingredients, toss, leave aside for 10 minutes, divide into smaller bowls and serve for breakfast.

Nutrition facts per serving: calories 161, fat 3, fiber 5, carbs 11, protein 7

Spinach and Eggs Mix

Prep time: 5 minutes I **Cooking time:** 25 minutes I **Servings:** 4

Ingredients:
- 8 eggs, whisked
- ½ cup almond milk
- 1 yellow onion, chopped
- 1 tablespoon olive oil
- 1 red bell pepper, chopped
- 1 yellow bell pepper, chopped
- 1 green bell pepper, chopped
- 2 cups baby spinach
- 1 tablespoon chives, chopped
- A pinch of salt and black pepper

Directions:
1. Heat up a pan with the oil over medium-high heat, add the onion, stir and sauté for 2 minutes.
2. Add the bell peppers, stir and cook for 3 minutes more.
3. Add the eggs whisked with the milk and the other ingredients, toss, spread into the pan, introduce it in the oven and cook at 360 degrees F for 20 minutes.
4. Divide it between plates and serve.

Nutrition facts per serving: calories 200, fat 3, fiber 6, carbs 14, protein 6

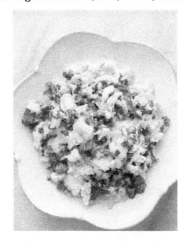

Pancakes

Prep time: 10 minutes I **Cooking time:** 10 minutes I **Servings:** 4

Ingredients:
- 2 eggs, whisked
- 1 teaspoon almond extract
- 1 cup almond milk
- 2 tablespoons almonds, chopped
- 1 cup almond flour
- 2 tablespoons coconut oil, melted

Directions:
1. In a bowl, combine the eggs with the almond extract, the milk, almonds, flour and 1 tablespoon oil, and stir really well.
2. Heat up a pan with the rest of the oil over medium heat, ¼ of the batter, spread into the pan, cook for 3 minutes on each side and transfer to a plate.
3. Repeat with the rest of the batter and serve the pancakes for breakfast.

Nutrition facts per serving: calories 121, fat 3, fiber 6, carbs 14, protein 6

Veggie Muffins

Prep time: 10 minutes I **Cooking time:** 20 minutes I **Servings:** 8

Ingredients:
- ¼ cup coconut oil, melted
- 3 eggs, whisked
- ½ teaspoon vanilla extract
- 1 teaspoon baking powder
- 1 cup mushrooms, sliced
- ½ cup almond flour
- Cooking spray

Directions:
1. In a bowl, combine the eggs with the oil and the other ingredients, and stir well.
2. Grease a muffin tray with cooking spray, divide the mushroom mix, introduce in the oven and bake at 350 degrees F for 20 minutes.
3. Divide the muffins between plates and serve for breakfast.

Nutrition facts per serving: calories 167, fat 4, fiber 7, carbs 15, protein 6

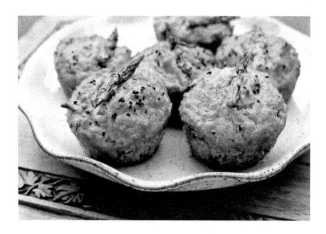

Almond Green Eggs

Prep time: 5 minutes I **Cooking time:** 14 minutes I **Servings:** 4

Ingredients:
- 1 cup baby kale
- 8 eggs, whisked
- ½ cup almond milk
- 2 spring onions, chopped
- 1 tablespoon olive oil
- 1 tablespoon cilantro, chopped
- A pinch of salt and black pepper

Directions:
1. Heat up a pan with the oil over medium heat, add the onions and sauté for 2 minutes.
2. Add the eggs mixed with the milk and the other ingredients, whisk, cook for 12 minutes more, divide between plates and serve.

Nutrition facts per serving: calories 176, fat 4, fiber 7, carbs 15, protein 7

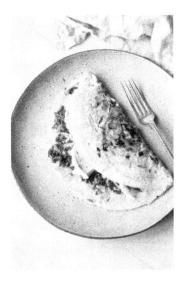

Honey Apple Bowls

Prep time: 5 minutes I **Cooking time:** 0 minutes I **Servings:** 4

Ingredients:
- 2 apples, peeled, cored and cubed
- 1 tablespoon pepitas
- 3 tablespoons flax seeds
- 1 cup water
- 2 cups coconut milk
- 2 tablespoons mint, chopped
- 3 tablespoons raw honey

Directions:
1. In a blender, combine the apples with the pepitas and the other ingredients, pulse well, divide into bowls and serve for breakfast.

Nutrition facts per serving: calories 171, fat 2, fiber 6, carbs 14, protein 5

Peppers and Olives Bowls

Prep time: 10 minutes I **Cooking time:** 0 minutes I **Servings:** 4

Ingredients:
- 1 red bell pepper, cut into strips
- 1 green bell pepper, cut into strips
- 2 spring onions, chopped
- 1 cup black olives, pitted and halved
- 1 cup kalamata olives, pitted and halved
- A pinch of garlic powder
- A pinch of salt and black pepper
- 1 tablespoon avocado oil

Directions:
1. In a bowl, combine the bell peppers with the onions and the other ingredients, toss, divide between plates and serve for breakfast.

Nutrition facts per serving: calories 221, fat 6, fiber 6, carbs 14, protein 11

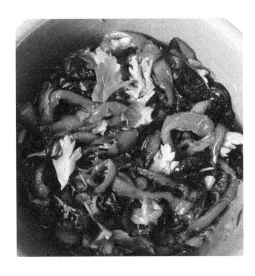

Chives Sweet Potato Mix

Prep time: 5 minutes I **Cooking time:** 15 minutes I **Servings:** 4

Ingredients:
- A pinch of salt and black pepper
- 8 eggs, whisked
- 1 tablespoon olive oil
- 1 small yellow onion, chopped
- 2 garlic cloves, minced
- 1 cup sweet potato, peeled and cubed
- 1 cup baby spinach
- 1 tablespoon chives, chopped

Directions:
1. Heat up a pan with the oil over medium-high heat, add the onion and the garlic and sauté for 2 minutes.
2. Add the potato, stir and cook for 3 minutes more.
3. Add the eggs and the other ingredients, cook for 10 minutes, stirring from time to time, divide between plates and serve for breakfast.

Nutrition facts per serving: calories 213.3, fat 12.3, fiber 7, carbs 14, protein 2.3

Avocado and Spinach Salad

Prep time: 5 minutes I **Cooking time:** 0 minutes I **Servings:** 2

Ingredients:
- 2 avocados, peeled, pitted and roughly cubed
- 1 mango, peeled and cubed
- 1 tablespoon lime juice
- 1 cup baby spinach
- A handful basil, torn
- 1 tablespoon olive oil
- ¼ cup pine nuts, toasted
- A pinch of salt and black pepper

Directions:
1. In a salad bowl, mix avocados with the mango and the other ingredients, toss and serve for breakfast.

Nutrition facts per serving: calories 200.1, fat 4, fiber 4, carbs 14.1, protein 5

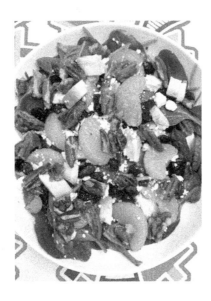

Turmeric Eggs and Sprouts

Prep time: 10 minutes I **Cooking time:** 15 minutes I **Servings:** 4

Ingredients:
- 1 cup Brussels sprouts, shredded
- 1 yellow onion, chopped
- 8 eggs, whisked
- 1 tablespoon olive oil
- 1 tablespoon turmeric powder
- 1 tablespoon cilantro, chopped
- 1 teaspoon cumin, ground
- A pinch of salt and black pepper

Directions:
1. Heat up a pan with the oil over medium-high heat, add the onion and the sprouts and sauté for 5 minutes.
2. Add the eggs and the other ingredients, toss well, cook for 10 minutes more, divide between plates and serve.

Nutrition facts per serving: calories 177, fat 2, fiber 6, carbs 15, protein 6

Lime Spinach Bowls

Prep time: 5 minutes I **Cooking time:** 0 minutes I **Servings:** 4

Ingredients:
- 2 cups baby spinach
- 10 strawberries, halved
- 1 tablespoon pine nuts
- 1 tablespoon almonds, chopped
- 1 tablespoon lime juice
- 1 tablespoon avocado oil

Directions:
1. In a bowl, combine the spinach with the strawberries and the other ingredients, toss and serve for breakfast.

Nutrition facts per serving: calories 171, fat 3, fiber 6, carbs 15, protein 5

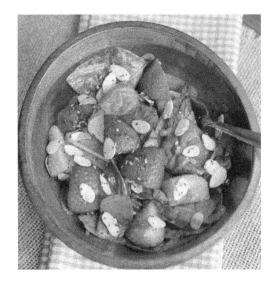

Spinach and Collard Greens Bowls

Prep time: 10 minutes I **Cooking time:** 20 minutes I **Servings:** 4

Ingredients:
- 1 cup old-fashioned oats
- 1 cup almond milk
- ½ cup water
- 1 tablespoon coconut oil, melted
- ½ cup collard greens, chopped
- ½ cup baby spinach, chopped
- A handful basil, chopped
- ½ tablespoon rosemary, chopped
- A pinch of salt and black pepper

Directions:
1. Heat up a pot with the milk and the water over medium heat, add the oats, the oil, and the other ingredients, cook for 20 minutes, stirring often, divide into bowls and serve warm.

Nutrition facts per serving: calories 246, fat 19.3, fiber 3.8, carbs 17.6, protein 4.1

Quinoa and Eggs Bowls

Prep time: 10 minutes I **Cooking time:** 0 minutes I **Servings:** 4

Ingredients:
- 1 cup baby spinach
- 1 cup baby kale
- 2 spring onions, chopped
- 2 tablespoons olive oil
- 1 cup quinoa, cooked
- 1 carrot, shredded
- 1 red bell pepper, cut into strips
- A pinch of salt and black pepper
- 1 tablespoon lime juice
- 4 eggs, hard boiled, peeled and roughly cubed

Directions:
1. In a salad bowl, combine the quinoa with the spinach, kale and the other ingredients, toss and serve for breakfast.

Nutrition facts per serving: calories 308, fat 14.1, fiber 4.4, carbs 34, protein 12.8

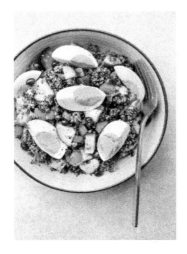

Barley and Kale Salad

Prep time: 10 minutes I **Cooking time:** 1 hour I **Servings:** 2

Ingredients:
- 1 cup black barley
- 3 cups water
- 2 fennel bulbs, shaved
- 1 cup baby kale
- 1 small red onion, sliced
- 2 tablespoons almonds, chopped
- 1 avocado, peeled, pitted and cubed
- 2 tablespoons oil
- 1 tablespoon pine nuts
- 2 tablespoons balsamic vinegar
- A pinch of salt and black pepper

Directions:
1. Put the barley in a pot, add the water, salt and pepper, bring to a simmer over medium heat, cook for 1 hour, drain, cool and transfer to a salad bowl.
2. Add the fennel, kale and the other ingredients, toss, divide into smaller bowls and serve for breakfast.

Nutrition facts per serving: calories 545, fat 41.2, fiber 18.1, carbs 42.7, protein 9.8

Sweet Potato and Carrots Mix

Prep time: 5 minutes I **Cooking time:** 20 minutes I **Servings:** 4

Ingredients:
- 2 scallions, chopped
- 2 tablespoons olive oil
- 4 sweet potatoes, peeled and cut into wedges
- 1 teaspoon chili powder
- 1 teaspoon hot paprika
- 2 carrots, shredded
- 1 teaspoon sesame seeds
- 1 tablespoon lime juice
- A pinch of salt and black pepper

Directions:
1. Heat up a pan with the oil over medium heat, add the scallions and sauté for 2 minutes.
2. Add the sweet potatoes and the other ingredients, toss, cook for 18 minutes more, divide into bowls and serve for breakfast.

Nutrition facts per serving: calories 371, fat 12.2, fiber 6, carbs 13.1, protein 5

Cucumber and Basil Mix

Prep time: 5 minutes I **Cooking time:** 0 minutes I **Servings:** 4

Ingredients:
- 2 tablespoons olive oil
- 2 scallions, chopped
- 1 tablespoon lime juice
- 1 tablespoon dill, chopped
- 3 cucumbers, roughly cubed
- 2 tablespoons chives, chopped
- 1 jalapeno, chopped
- A handful basil, chopped
- 1 tablespoon almonds, crushed
- 1 tablespoon walnuts, chopped
- A pinch of salt and black pepper

Directions:
1. In a salad bowl, combine the cucumbers with the scallions and the other ingredients, toss, divide into smaller bowls and serve for breakfast.

Nutrition facts per serving: calories 199, fat 4, fiber 8, carbs 15, protein 4

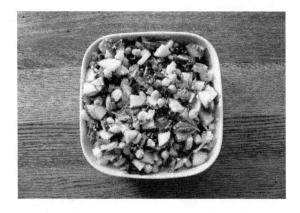

Zucchinis and Arugula Bowls

Prep time: 10 minutes I **Cooking time:** 0 minutes I **Servings:** 4

Ingredients:
- 2 zucchinis, cut with a spiralizer
- 1 cup barley, cooked
- 2 scallions, chopped
- 1 tablespoon olive oil
- ½ teaspoon sweet paprika
- A pinch of chili powder
- 1 tablespoon lime juice
- A pinch of salt and black pepper
- 1 tablespoon oregano, chopped
- 2 cups baby arugula
- ½ cup sesame seeds paste
- 1 tablespoon balsamic vinegar
- 1 garlic clove, minced
- ½ teaspoon cumin, ground

Directions:
1. In a large bowl, combine the zucchinis with the barley, scallions and the other ingredients, toss, divide between plates and serve for breakfast.

Nutrition facts per serving: calories 226, fat 5, fiber 7, carbs 16, protein 7

Eggs and Scallions Mix

Prep time: 10 minutes I **Cooking time:** 15 minutes I **Servings:** 4

Ingredients:
- 1 avocado, peeled, pitted and cubed
- 6 eggs, whisked
- 2 scallions, chopped
- 1 red bell pepper, chopped
- 2 tablespoons olive oil
- 2 garlic cloves, minced
- 2 eggs, whisked
- 1 tablespoon cilantro, chopped

Directions:
1. Heat up a pan with the oil over medium-high heat, add the scallions, garlic and the bell pepper and sauté for 5 minutes.
2. Add the avocado and the other ingredients, toss, cook for 10 minutes over medium heat, divide between plates and serve.

Nutrition facts per serving: calories 211, fat 2, fiber 5, carbs 16, protein 5

Almond Frittata

Prep time: 10 minutes I **Cooking time:** 20 minutes I **Servings:** 4

Ingredients:
- 8 eggs, whisked
- 2 shallots, chopped
- 1 cup kalamata olives, pitted and chopped
- 1 tablespoon coriander, chopped
- 1 tablespoon chives, chopped
- 1 tablespoon olive oil
- 1 cup almond milk
- A pinch of salt and black pepper

Directions:
1. Heat up a pan with the oil over medium heat, add the shallots and sauté for 2 minutes.
2. Add the eggs mixed with the milk and the other ingredients, toss, spread into the pan, introduce the frittata in the oven and cook at 360 degrees F for 18 minutes.
3. Divide the frittata between plates and serve.

Nutrition facts per serving: calories 201, fat 6, fiber 9, carbs 14, protein 6

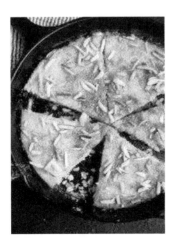

Blueberries Bowls

Prep time: 10 minutes I **Cooking time:** 15 minutes I **Servings:** 4

Ingredients:
- 1 cup blueberries
- 1 tablespoon coconut oil, melted
- 1/3 cup coconut flakes
- 1 cup coconut milk
- ½ teaspoon nutmeg, ground
- ½ teaspoon vanilla extract

Directions:
1. In a small pot, mix the berries with the oil and the other ingredients, toss, simmer over medium heat for 15 minutes, divide into bowls and serve.

Nutrition facts per serving: calories 208, fat 2, fiber 6, carbs 16, protein 8

Balsamic Spinach Salad

Prep time: 5 minutes I **Cooking time:** 0 minutes I **Servings:** 4

Ingredients:
- 2 cups baby spinach, torn
- 2 shallots, chopped
- 1 cup cucumber, cubed
- 1 cup kalamata olives, pitted and sliced
- 1 tablespoon chives, chopped
- 1 tablespoon balsamic vinegar
- A pinch of salt and black pepper
- 2 tablespoons olive oil

Directions:
1. In a salad bowl, mix the spinach with the shallots, the cucumber and the other ingredients, toss, divide between plates and serve for breakfast.

Nutrition facts per serving: calories 171, fat 2, fiber 5, carbs 11, protein 5

Parsley Potato Bowls

Prep time: 5 minutes I **Cooking time:** 20 minutes I **Servings:** 4

Ingredients:
- 2 sweet potatoes, peeled and cubed
- 1 cup coconut cream
- 3 garlic cloves, minced
- 2 tablespoons olive oil
- 1 yellow onion, chopped
- 1 teaspoon cumin, ground
- 1 teaspoon turmeric powder
- 2 tablespoons parsley, chopped
- A pinch of salt and black pepper

Directions:
1. Heat up a pan with the oil over medium-high heat, add the onion, garlic, cumin and turmeric, stir and sauté for 5 minutes.
2. Add the potatoes and the other ingredients, toss, cook for 15 minutes more, divide into bowls and serve for breakfast.

Nutrition facts per serving: calories 188, fat 2, fiber 8, carbs 10, protein 4

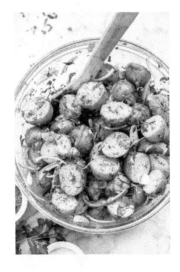

Parsley Eggs

Prep time: 10 minutes I **Cooking time:** 12 minutes I **Servings:** 4

Ingredients:

- 8 eggs, whisked
- 2 shallots, chopped
- A pinch of salt and black pepper
- 1 cucumber, cubed
- 1 tablespoon parsley, chopped
- 1 tablespoon olive oil

Directions:

1. Heat up a pan with the oil over medium-high heat, add the shallots and sauté for 2 minutes.
2. Add the eggs mixed with the other ingredients, toss, spread into the pan, cook for 5 minutes, flip and cook for another 5 minutes.
3. Cut the omelet, divide it between plates and serve for breakfast.

Nutrition facts per serving: calories 201, fat 2, fiber 5, carbs 11, protein 5

Coconut Maple Oatmeal

Prep time: 10 minutes I **Cooking time:** 20 minutes I **Servings:** 4

Ingredients:
- 2 cups coconut milk
- 1 cup old fashioned oats
- 2 tablespoons flax meal
- 1 teaspoon vanilla extract
- 2 teaspoons cinnamon powder
- 1 teaspoon maple syrup

Directions:
1. In a small pot, mix the oats with the milk and the other ingredients, toss, bring to a simmer, cook over medium heat for 20 minutes, divide into bowls and serve for breakfast.

Nutrition facts per serving: calories 454, fat 32.4, fiber 7.6, carbs 35.7, protein 8.5

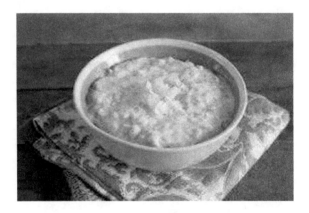

Coconut Broccoli Mix

Prep time: 10 minutes I **Cooking time:** 15 minutes I **Servings:** 4

Ingredients:
- 1 pound broccoli florets
- 1 yellow onion, chopped
- 1 tablespoon olive oil
- ½ cup coconut cream
- 1 teaspoon chili powder
- 1 teaspoon hot paprika
- 1 teaspoon garlic powder
- A pinch of salt and black pepper

Directions:
1. Heat up a pan with the oil over medium-high heat, add the onion and sauté for 2 minutes.
2. Add the rest of the ingredients, toss, cook for 12 minutes over medium heat, divide into bowls and serve for breakfast.

Nutrition facts per serving: calories 153, fat 11.2, fiber 4.5, carbs 12.7, protein 4.4

Green Olives Bowls

Prep time: 5 minutes I **Cooking time:** 0 minutes I **Servings:** 4

Ingredients:
- 1 cup spinach, torn
- 1 cup kale, torn
- 1 cup black olives, pitted and halved
- 2 shallots, chopped
- 1 tablespoon lemon juice
- 1 tablespoon avocado oil
- 1 tablespoon mint, chopped

Directions:
1. In a bowl, mix the spinach with the kale and the other ingredients, toss, and serve for breakfast.

Nutrition facts per serving: calories 198, fat 6.4, fiber 2, carbs 8, protein 6

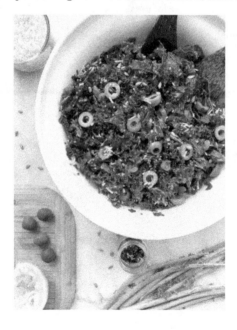

Tomato and Spring Onions Salad

Prep time: 6 minutes I **Cooking time:** 0 minutes I **Servings:** 4

Ingredients:
- 1 cup cherry tomatoes, halved
- 2 oranges, peeled and cut into segments
- 3 spring onions, chopped
- 1 tablespoon olive oil
- 1 tablespoon lemon juice
- A pinch of salt and black pepper
- 1 teaspoon turmeric powder

Directions:
1. In a bowl, mix the tomatoes with the oranges and the other ingredients, toss and serve for breakfast.

Nutrition facts per serving: calories 255, fat 4, fiber 5, carbs 15, protein 6

Citrus Pear Salad

Prep time: 10 minutes I **Cooking time:** 15 minutes I **Servings:** 4

Ingredients:
- 2 cups pears, cored and cubed
- 1/3 cup coconut flakes, unsweetened
- 2 tablespoons orange juice
- 1 cup baby kale
- 1 tablespoon avocado oil

Directions:
1. In a bowl, combine the pears with the coconut and the other ingredients, toss and serve for breakfast.

Nutrition facts per serving: calories 172, fat 5, fiber 7, carbs 8, protein 4

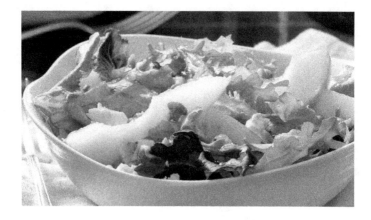

Cantaloupe Bowls

Prep time: 5 minutes I **Cooking time:** 0 minutes I **Servings:** 2

Ingredients:
- 2 tablespoons walnuts, chopped
- 1 cup blackberries
- 1 cup cantaloupe, peeled and cubed
- 1 tablespoon lime juice
- 1 tablespoon orange juice
- 1 teaspoon vanilla extract

Directions:
1. In a bowl, mix the blackberries with the walnuts and other ingredients, toss, divide into smaller bowls and serve for breakfast.

Nutrition facts per serving: calories 90, fat 0.3, fiber 1, carbs 0, protein 5

Cauliflower and Eggs Pan

Prep time: 5 minutes I **Cooking time:** 20 minutes I **Servings:** 4

Ingredients:
- 1 cup cauliflower florets
- 1 small sweet onion, chopped
- 1 tablespoon olive oil
- 1 tablespoon lemon juice
- 1 teaspoon turmeric powder
- 1 teaspoon cumin, ground
- 2 garlic cloves, minced
- Salt and black pepper to the taste
- 4 eggs

Directions:
1. Heat up a pan with the oil over medium-high heat, add the onion, and the garlic, stir and sauté for 5 minutes.
2. Add the cauliflower and cook for 5 minutes more.
3. Add the rest of the ingredients, toss, cook for 10 minutes more, divide into bowls and serve.

Nutrition facts per serving: calories 214, fat 7, fiber 2, carbs 12, protein 8

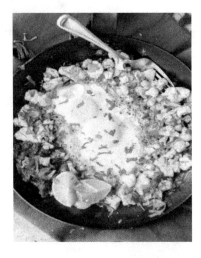

Berries and Walnuts Oats

Prep time: 10 minutes I **Cooking time:** 20 minutes I **Servings:** 4

Ingredients:
- 2 tablespoons walnuts, chopped
- 1 tablespoon almonds, chopped
- 1 cup cranberries
- 2 cups almond milk
- ½ cup old fashioned oats
- 1 teaspoon vanilla extract
- 1 teaspoon cinnamon powder

Directions:
1. In a small pot, combine the cranberries with the oats, the milk and the other ingredients, toss, bring to a simmer and cook for 20 minutes.
2. Divide the mix into bowls and serve for breakfast.

Nutrition facts per serving: calories 190, fat 1, fiber 1, carbs 7, protein 6

Spinach and Avocado Smoothie

Prep time: 5 minutes I **Cooking time:** 0 minutes I **Servings:** 4

Ingredients:
- 2 avocados, pitted, peeled and chopped
- 1 banana, frozen, peeled and roughly chopped
- 2 cups baby spinach
- 1 tablespoon almonds, chopped
- 2 cups almond milk, unsweetened

Directions:
1. In your blender, mix the avocados with the spinach and the other ingredients, pulse well, divide into bowls and serve for breakfast.

Nutrition facts per serving: calories 519, fat 49.1, fiber 10.7, carbs 22.9, protein 5.7

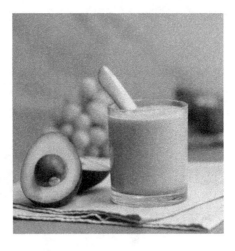

Arugula, Beets and Tomato Salad

Prep time: 5 minutes I **Cooking time:** 0 minutes I **Servings:** 4

Ingredients:
- 2 cups beets, baked, peeled and cubed
- 1 cup baby arugula
- 2 tablespoons olive oil
- 2 shallots, chopped
- 1 cup cherry tomatoes, halved
- Juice of 1 lime
- ¼ inch ginger, grated

Directions:
1. In a salad bowl, mix the beets with the arugula and the other ingredients, toss, divide into smaller bowls and serve for breakfast.

Nutrition facts per serving: calories 114, fat 7.3, fiber 2.4, carbs 12/4, protein 2.2

Quinoa Bowls

Prep time: 5 minutes I **Cooking time:** 0 minutes I **Servings:** 4

Ingredients:
- 2 cups quinoa, cooked
- 1 cup strawberries, halved
- 1 tablespoon maple syrup
- ½ tablespoon lime juice
- 1 teaspoon vanilla extract

Directions:
1. In a bowl, mix the quinoa with the strawberries and the other ingredients, toss, divide into smaller bowls and serve for breakfast.

Nutrition facts per serving: calories 170, fat 5.3, fiber 6, carbs 6.8, protein 5

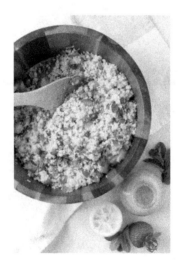

Carrots and Quinoa Mix

Prep time: 5 minutes I **Cooking time:** 10 minutes I **Servings:** 4

Ingredients:
- 2 tablespoon maple syrup
- 1 tablespoon almonds, chopped
- 2 cups carrots, shredded
- 1 cup quinoa, cooked
- ¼ teaspoon turmeric powder
- 2 tablespoons sesame seeds
- 1 tablespoon lime juice

Directions:
1. In a salad bowl, combine the carrots with the quinoa and the other ingredients, toss, divide into ramekins, cook at 350 degrees F for 10 minutes and serve for breakfast.

Nutrition facts per serving: calories 150, fat 3, fiber 2, carbs 6, protein 8

Tomato and Scallions Salad

Prep time: 5 minutes I **Cooking time:** 0 minutes I **Servings:** 4

Ingredients:
- 2 cups cherry tomatoes, halved
- 2 scallions, chopped
- 1 tablespoon basil, chopped
- 1 avocado, peeled, pitted and cubed
- 2 tablespoons oregano, chopped
- 1 tablespoon mint, chopped
- 2 tablespoons balsamic vinegar
- 2 tablespoons olive oil
- A pinch of salt and black pepper

Directions:
1. In a salad bowl, mix the tomatoes with the scallions, the basil and the other ingredients, toss, divide into smaller bowls and serve for breakfast.

Nutrition facts per serving: calories 140, fat 2, fiber 3, carbs 6, protein 8

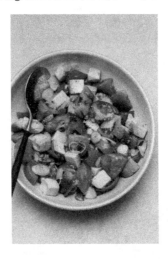

Black Beans Mix

Prep time: 5 minutes I **Cooking time:** 15 minutes I **Servings:** 4

Ingredients:
- 1 cup black beans, cooked
- 2 green onions, chopped
- 6 eggs, whisked
- ½ teaspoon cumin, ground
- 1 teaspoon chili powder
- 2 scallions, chopped
- 1 tablespoon olive oil
- ½ cup cilantro, chopped
- 2 tablespoons pine nuts
- A pinch of salt and black pepper

Directions:
1. Heat up a pan with the oil over medium heat, add the scallions, green onions and pine nuts, stir and cook for 2 minutes.
2. Add the beans and cook them for 3 minutes more.
3. Add the eggs and the rest of the ingredients and cook for 10 minutes more, stirring often.
4. Divide everything between plates and serve for breakfast.

Nutrition facts per serving: calories 140, fat 4, fiber 2, carbs 7, protein 8

Onion, Corn and Avocado Salad

Prep time: 5 minutes I **Cooking time:** 0 minutes I **Servings:** 4

Ingredients:
- 2 avocados, pitted, peeled and cubed
- 1 cup corn
- 2 spring onions, chopped
- 2 red bell peppers, roughly chopped
- 2 tablespoons olive oil
- 1 tablespoon lime juice
- A pinch of salt and black pepper
- 1 tablespoon chives, chopped

Directions:
1. In a salad bowl, mix the corn with the avocado and the other ingredients, toss well, divide into smaller bowls and serve for breakfast.

Nutrition facts per serving: calories 140, fat 3, fiber 2, carbs 6, protein 9

Basil Eggs

Prep time: 5 minutes I **Cooking time:** 15 minutes I **Servings:** 4

Ingredients:
- 2 tablespoons extra-virgin olive oil
- 1 yellow onion, chopped
- 1 cup cherry tomatoes, quartered
- 6 eggs, whisked
- 1 tablespoon basil, chopped
- A pinch of salt and black pepper

Directions:
1. Heat up a pan with the oil over medium-high heat, add the onion and sauté for 5 minutes.
2. Add the eggs and the remaining ingredients, toss, cook for 10 minutes more, divide between plates and serve.

Nutrition facts per serving: calories 100, fat 1, fiber 2, carbs 2, protein 6

Zucchini Spread

Prep time: 10 minutes I **Cooking time:** 15 minutes I **Servings:** 4

Ingredients:
- 1 pound zucchini, chopped
- 1 yellow onion, chopped
- 1 tablespoon coconut cream
- ¼ cup veggie stock
- 2 tablespoons olive oil
- 2 tablespoons lemon juice
- ¼ cup parsley, chopped
- A pinch of salt and black pepper

Directions:
1. Heat up a pan with the oil over medium heat, add the onion, stir and cook for 2 minutes.
2. Add the zucchinis and the other ingredients, stir, bring to a simmer, cook for 13 minutes more, blend using an immersion blender, divide into bowls and serve as a morning spread.

Nutrition facts per serving: calories 102, fat 8.3, fiber 2.1, carbs 7.1, protein 1.9

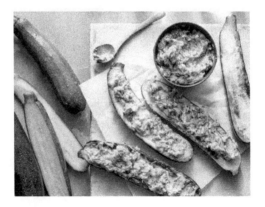

Watermelon Salad

Prep time: 10 minutes I **Cooking time:** 0 minutes I **Servings:** 4

Ingredients:
- ½ teaspoon maple syrup
- 2 tablespoons lemon juice
- 1 tablespoon avocado oil
- 1 cup watermelon, peeled and cubed
- 1 cup baby arugula
- 1 cup quinoa, cooked
- ½ cup basil leaves, chopped

Directions:
1. In a bowl, mix the watermelon with the arugula and the other ingredients, toss and serve for breakfast.

Nutrition facts per serving: calories 179, fat 3.2, fiber 3.4, carbs 31.3, protein 6.5

Mango Coconut Oatmeal

Prep time: 10 minutes I **Cooking time:** 20 minutes I **Servings:** 4

Ingredients:
- 2 cups coconut milk
- 1 cup old-fashioned oats
- 1 cup mango, peeled and cubed
- 3 tablespoons almond butter
- 2 tablespoons coconut sugar
- ½ teaspoon vanilla extract

Directions:
1. Put the milk in a pot, heat it up over medium heat, add the oats and the other ingredients, stir, bring to a simmer and cook for 20 minutes.
2. Stir the oatmeal, divide it into bowls and serve.

Nutrition facts per serving: calories 531, fat 41.8, fiber 7.5, carbs 42.7, protein 9.3

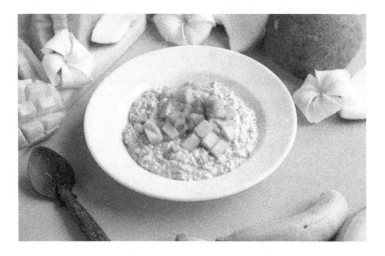

Cherries Oats

Prep time: 10 minutes I **Cooking time:** 10 minutes I **Servings:** 6

Ingredients:
- 2 cups old-fashioned oats
- 3 cups almond milk
- 2 and ½ tablespoons cocoa powder
- 1 teaspoon vanilla extract
- 10 ounces cherries, pitted
- 2 pears, cored, peeled and cubed

Directions:
1. In your pressure cooker, combine the oats with the milk and the other ingredients, toss, cover and cook on High for 10 minutes.
2. Release the pressure naturally for 10 minutes, stir the oatmeal one more time, divide it into bowls and serve.

Nutrition facts per serving: calories 477, fat 30.7, fiber 8.3, carbs 49.6, protein 7

Pecan Oats

Prep time: 10 minutes I **Cooking time:** 20 minutes I **Servings:** 4

Ingredients:
- 1 cup steel cut oats
- 2 cups orange juice
- 2 tablespoons coconut butter, melted
- 2 tablespoons stevia
- 3 tablespoons pecans, chopped
- ¼ teaspoon vanilla extract

Directions:
1. Heat up a pot with the orange juice over medium heat, add the oats, the butter and the other ingredients, whisk, simmer for 20 minutes, divide into bowls and serve for breakfast.

Nutrition facts per serving: calories 288, fat 39.1, fiber 3.4, carbs 48.3, protein 4.7

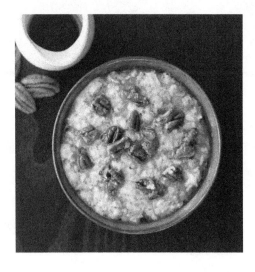

Creamy Peaches

Prep time: 10 minutes I **Cooking time:** 20 minutes I **Servings:** 4

Ingredients:
- 2 cups coconut cream
- 1 teaspoon cinnamon powder
- 1/3 cup palm sugar
- 4 peaches, stones removed and cut into wedges
- Cooking spray

Directions:
1. Grease a baking pan with the cooking spray and combine the peaches with the other ingredients inside.
2. Bake this at 360 degrees F for 20 minutes, divide into bowls and serve for breakfast.

Nutrition facts per serving: calories 338, fat 29.2, fiber 4.9, carbs 21, protein 4.2

Maple Yogurt Bowls

Prep time: 10 minutes I **Cooking time:** 15 minutes I **Servings:** 4

Ingredients:
- 1 cup steel cut oats
- 1 and ½ cups almond milk
- 1 cup non-fat yogurt
- ¼ cup maple syrup
- 2 apples, cored, peeled and chopped
- ½ teaspoon cinnamon powder

Directions:
1. In a pot, combine the oats with the m ilk and the other ingredients except the yogurt, toss, bring to a simmer and cook over medium-high heat for 15 minutes.
2. Divide the yogurt into bowls, divide the apples and oats mix on top and serve for breakfast.

Nutrition facts per serving: calories 490, fat 30.2, fiber 7.4, carbs 53.9, protein 7

Pomegranate Oatmeal

Prep time: 10 minutes I **Cooking time:** 20 minutes I **Servings:** 4

Ingredients:
- 3 cups almond milk
- 1 cup steel cut oats
- 1 tablespoon cinnamon powder
- 1 mango, peeled, and cubed
- ½ teaspoon vanilla extract
- 3 tablespoons pomegranate seeds

Directions:
1. Put the milk in a pot and heat it up over medium heat.
2. Add the oats, cinnamon and the other ingredients, toss, simmer for 20 minutes, divide into bowls and serve for breakfast.

Nutrition facts per serving: calories 568, fat 44.6, fiber 7.5, carbs 42.5, protein 7.8

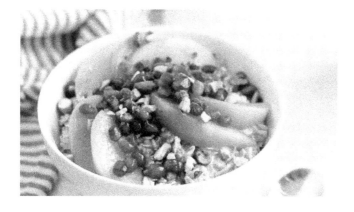

Chia Bowls

Prep time: 10 minutes I **Cooking time:** 20 minutes I **Servings:** 4

Ingredients:
- ½ cup steel cut oats
- 2 cups almond milk
- ¼ cup pomegranate seeds
- 4 tablespoons chia seeds
- 1 teaspoon vanilla extract

Directions:
1. Put the milk in a pot, bring to a simmer over medium heat, add the oats and the other ingredients, bring to a simmer and cook for 20 minutes.
2. Divide the mix into bowls and serve for breakfast.

Nutrition facts per serving: calories 462, fat 38, fiber 13.5, carbs 27.1, protein 8.8

Carrots Hash

Prep time: 10 minutes I **Cooking time:** 20 minutes I **Servings:** 4

Ingredients:
- 2 carrots, peeled and cubed
- 1 tablespoon olive oil
- 1 yellow onion, chopped
- 1 cup cheddar cheese, shredded
- 8 eggs, whisked
- 1 cup coconut milk
- A pinch of salt and black pepper

Directions:
1. Heat up a pan with the oil over medium heat, add the onion and the carrots, toss and brown for 5 minutes.
2. Add the eggs and the other ingredients, toss, cook for 15 minutes stirring often, divide between plates and serve.

Nutrition facts per serving: calories 431, fat 35.9, fiber 2.7, carbs 10, protein 20

Peppers and Eggs Mix

Prep time: 10 minutes I **Cooking time:** 15 minutes I **Servings:** 4

Ingredients:
- 4 eggs, whisked
- A pinch of black pepper
- ¼ cup bacon, chopped
- 1 tablespoon olive oil
- 1 cup red bell peppers, chopped
- 4 spring onions, chopped
- ¾ cup cheddar, shredded

Directions:
1. Heat up a pan with the oil over medium heat, add the spring onions and the bell peppers, toss and cook for 5 minutes.
2. Add the eggs and the other ingredients, toss, spread into the pan, cook for 5 minutes, flip, cook for another 5 minutes, divide between plates and serve.

Nutrition facts per serving: calories 288, fat 18, fiber 0.8, carbs 4, protein 13.4

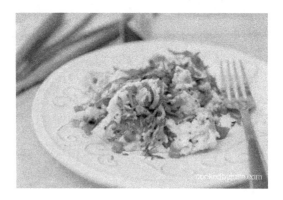

Parsley Eggs

Prep time: 10 minutes I **Cooking time:** 20 minutes I **Servings:** 4

Ingredients:
- A pinch of black pepper
- 4 eggs, whisked
- 2 tablespoons parsley, chopped
- 1 tablespoon cheddar cheese, shredded
- 1 red onion, chopped
- 1 tablespoon olive oil

Directions:
1. Heat up a pan with the oil over medium heat, add the onion and the black pepper, stir and sauté for 5 minutes.
2. Add the eggs mixed with the other ingredients, spread into the pan, introduce in the oven and cook at 360 degrees F for 15 minutes.
3. Divide the frittata between plates and serve.

Nutrition facts per serving: calories 112, fat 8.5, fiber 0.7, carb 3.1, protein 6.3

Artichoke Eggs Mix

Prep time: 5 minutes I **Cooking time:** 20 minutes I **Servings:** 4

Ingredients:
- 4 eggs
- 4 slices cheddar, shredded
- 1 yellow onion, chopped
- 1 tablespoon avocado oil
- 1 tablespoon cilantro, chopped
- 1 cup artichokes, chopped

Directions:
1. Grease 4 ramekins with the oil, divide the onion in each, crack an egg in each ramekin, add the artichokes and top with cilantro and cheddar cheese.
2. Introduce the ramekins in the oven and bake at 380 degrees F for 20 minutes.
3. Serve the baked eggs for breakfast.

Nutrition facts per serving: calories 178, fat 10.9, fiber 2.9, carbs 8.4, protein 14.2

Beans and Eggs

Prep time: 10 minutes I **Cooking time:** 30 minutes I **Servings:** 8

Ingredients:
- 8 eggs, whisked
- 2 red onions, chopped
- 1 red bell pepper, chopped
- 4 ounces black beans, cooked
- ½ cup green onions, chopped
- 1 cup mozzarella cheese, shredded
- Cooking spray

Directions:
1. Grease a baking pan with the cooking spray and spread the black beans, onions, green onions and bell pepper into the pan.
2. Add the eggs mixed with the cheese, introduce in the oven and bake at 380 degrees F for 30 minutes.
3. Divide the mix between plates and serve for breakfast.

Nutrition facts per serving: calories 140, fat 4.7, fiber 3.4, carbs 13.6, protein 11.2

Mozzarella Scramble

Prep time: 10 minutes I **Cooking time:** 15 minutes I **Servings:** 4

Ingredients:
- 3 tablespoons mozzarella, shredded
- A pinch of black pepper
- 4 eggs, whisked
- 1 red bell pepper, chopped
- 1 teaspoon turmeric powder
- 1 tablespoon olive oil
- 2 shallots, chopped

Directions:
1. Heat up a pan with the oil over medium heat, add the shallots and the bell pepper, stir and sauté for 5 minutes.
2. Add the eggs mixed with the rest of the ingredients, stir, cook for 10 minutes, divide everything between plates and serve.

Nutrition facts per serving: calories 138, fat 8, fiber 1.3, carbs 4.6, protein 12

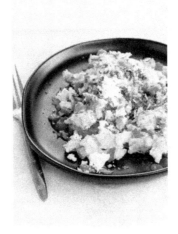

Cheddar Hash Browns

Prep time: 10 minutes I **Cooking time:** 20 minutes I **Servings:** 4

Ingredients:
- 1 tablespoon olive oil
- 4 eggs, whisked
- 1 cup hash browns
- ½ cup cheddar cheese, shredded
- 1 small yellow onion, chopped
- A pinch of black pepper
- ½ green bell pepper, chopped
- ½ red bell pepper, chopped
- 1 carrot, chopped
- 1 tablespoon cilantro, chopped

Directions:
1. Heat up a pan with the oil over medium-high heat, add the onion and the hash browns and cook for 5 minutes.
2. Add the bell peppers and the carrots, toss and cook for 5 minutes more.
3. Add the eggs, black pepper and the cheese, stir and cook for another 10 minutes.
4. Add the cilantro, stir, cook for a couple more seconds, divide everything between plates and serve for breakfast.

Nutrition facts per serving: calories 277, fat 17.5, fiber 2.7, carbs 19.9, protein 11

Chives Rice Mix

Prep time: 10 minutes I **Cooking time:** 25 minutes I **Servings:** 4

Ingredients:
- 3 slices bacon, chopped
- 1 tablespoon avocado oil
- 1 cup brown rice
- 1 red onion, chopped
- 2 cups chicken stock
- 2 tablespoons parmesan, grated
- 1 tablespoon chives, chopped
- A pinch of black pepper

Directions:
1. Heat up a pan with the oil over medium-high heat, add the onion and the bacon, stir and cook for 5 minutes.
2. Add the rice and the other ingredients, toss, bring to a simmer and cook over medium heat for 20 minutes.
3. Stir the mix, divide into bowls and serve for breakfast.

Nutrition facts per serving: calories 271, fat 7.2, fiber 1.4, carbs 40, protein 9.9

Cinnamon Quinoa

Prep time: 5 minutes I **Cooking time:** 10 minutes I **Servings:** 4

Ingredients:
- 1 and ½ cups water
- 1 teaspoon cinnamon powder
- 1 and ½ cups quinoa
- 1 cup almond milk
- 1 tablespoon coconut sugar
- ¼ cup pistachios, chopped

Directions:
1. Put the water and the almond milk in a pot, bring to a boil over medium heat, add the quinoa and the other ingredients, whisk, cook for 10 minutes, divide in to bowls, cool down and serve for breakfast.

Nutrition facts per serving: calories 222, fat 16.7, fiber 2.5, carbs 16.3, protein 3.9

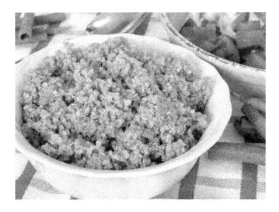

Cherries Mix

Prep time: 10 minutes I **Cooking time:** 0 minutes I **Servings:** 4

Ingredients:
- 4 cups non-fat yogurt
- 1 cup cherries, pitted and halved
- 4 tablespoons coconut sugar
- ½ teaspoon vanilla extract

Directions:
1. In a bowl, combine the yogurt with the cherries, sugar and vanilla, toss and keep in the fridge for 10 minutes.
2. Divide into bowls and serve f breakfast.

Nutrition facts per serving: calories 145, fat 0, fiber 0.1, carbs 29, protein 2.3

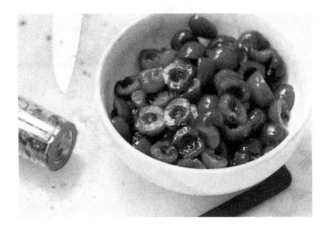

Plum and Sunflower Mix

Prep time: 10 minutes I **Cooking time:** 15 minutes I **Servings:** 4

Ingredients:
- 4 plums, pitted and halved
- 3 tablespoons coconut oil, melted
- ½ teaspoon cinnamon powder
- 1 cup coconut cream
- ¼ cup unsweetened coconut, shredded
- 2 tablespoons sunflower seeds, toasted

Directions:
1. In a baking dish, combine the plums with the oil, cinnamon and the other ingredients, introduce in the oven and bake at 380 degrees F for 15 minutes.
2. Divide everything into bowls and serve.

Nutrition facts per serving: calories 282, fat 27.1, fiber 2.8, carbs 12.4, protein 2.3

Apples and Cinnamon Yogurt

Prep time: 10 minutes I **Cooking time:** 0 minutes I **Servings:** 4

Ingredients:
- 6 apples, cored and pureed
- 1 cup natural apple juice
- 2 tablespoons coconut sugar
- 2 cups non-fat yogurt
- 1 teaspoon cinnamon powder

Directions:
1. In a bowl, combine the apples with the apple juice and the other ingredients, stir, divide into bowls and keep in the fridge for 10 minutes before serving.

Nutrition facts per serving: calories 289, fat 0.6, fiber 8.7, carbs 68.5, protein 3.9

Almond Strawberry Bowls

Prep time: 10 minutes I **Cooking time:** 20 minutes I **Servings:** 4

Ingredients:
- 1 and ½ cups gluten-free oats
- 2 and ¼ cups almond milk
- ½ teaspoon vanilla extract
- 2 cups strawberries, sliced
- 2 tablespoons coconut sugar

Directions:
1. Put the milk in a pot, bring to a simmer over medium heat, add the oats and the other ingredients, stir, cook for 20 minutes, divide into bowls and serve for breakfast.

Nutrition facts per serving: calories 216, fat 1.5, fiber 3.4, carbs 39.5, protein 10.4

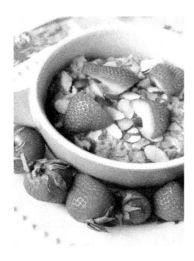

Almond Peach Mix

Prep time: 10 minutes I **Cooking time:** 15 minutes I **Servings:** 4

Ingredients:
- 4 peaches, cored and cut into wedges
- ¼ cup maple syrup
- ¼ teaspoon almond extract
- ½ cup almond milk

Directions:
1. Put the almond milk in a pot, bring to a simmer over medium heat, add the peaches and the other ingredients, toss, cook for 15 minutes, divide into bowls and serve for breakfast.

Nutrition facts per serving: calories 180, fat 7.6, fiber 3, carbs 28.9, protein 2.1

Almond Rice

Prep time: 10 minutes I **Cooking time:** 20 minutes I **Servings:** 4

Ingredients:
- 1 cup brown rice
- 2 cups almond milk
- 4 dates, chopped
- 2 tablespoons cinnamon powder
- 2 tablespoons coconut sugar

Directions:
1. In a pot, combine the rice with the milk and the other ingredients, bring to a simmer and cook over medium heat for 20 minutes.
2. Stir the mix again, divide into bowls and serve for breakfast.

Nutrition facts per serving: calories 516, fat 29, fiber 3.9, carbs 59.4, protein 6.8

Figs Yogurt

Prep time: 10 minutes I **Cooking time:** 0 minutes I **Servings:** 4

Ingredients:
- 1 cup figs, halved
- 1 pear, cored and cubed
- ½ cup pomegranate seeds
- ½ cup coconut sugar
- 2 cups non-fat yogurt

Directions:
1. In a bowl, combine the figs with the yogurt and the other ingredients, toss, divide into bowls and serve for breakfast.

Nutrition facts per serving: calories 223, fat 0.5, fiber 6.1, carbs 52, protein 4.5

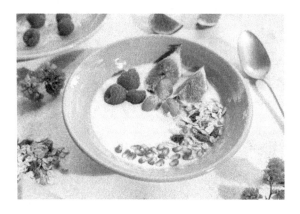

Coconut Porridge

Prep time: 10 minutes I **Cooking time:** 20 minutes I **Servings:** 4

Ingredients:
- 4 cups coconut milk
- 1 cup cornmeal
- 1 teaspoon vanilla extract
- 1 cup strawberries, halved
- ½ teaspoon nutmeg, ground

Directions:
1. Put the milk in a pot, bring to a simmer over medium heat, add the cornmeal and the other ingredients, toss, cook for 20 minutes, and take off the heat.
2. Divide the porridge between plates and serve for breakfast.

Nutrition facts per serving: calories 678, fat 58.5, fiber 8.3, carbs 39.8, protein 8.2

Brown Rice Mix

Prep time: 10 minutes I **Cooking time:** 20 minutes I **Servings:** 4

Ingredients:
- 1 cup brown rice
- 2 cups coconut milk
- 1 tablespoon cinnamon powder
- 1 cup blackberries
- ½ cup coconut cream, unsweetened

Directions:
1. Put the milk in a pot, bring to a simmer over medium heat, add the rice and the other ingredients, cook for 20 minutes, and divide into bowls.
2. Serve warm for breakfast.

Nutrition facts per serving: calories 469, fat 30.1, fiber 6.5, carbs 47.4, protein 7

Vanilla Rice

Prep time: 10 minutes I **Cooking time:** 20 minutes I **Servings:** 6

Ingredients:
- 2 cups coconut milk
- 1 cup basmati rice
- 2 tablespoons coconut sugar
- ¾ cup coconut cream
- 1 teaspoon vanilla extract

Directions:
1. In a pot, combine the milk with the rice and the other ingredients, stir, bring to a simmer and cook over medium heat for 20 minutes.
2. Stir the mix again, divide into bowls and serve for breakfast.

Nutrition facts per serving: calories 462, fat 25.3, fiber 2.2, carbs 55.2, protein 4.8

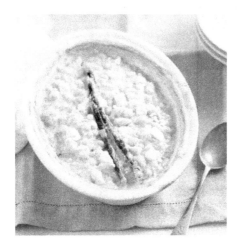

Cherries Rice

Prep time: 10 minutes I **Cooking time:** 25 minutes I **Servings:** 4

Ingredients:
- 1 tablespoon coconut, shredded
- 2 tablespoons coconut sugar
- 1 cup brown rice
- 2 cups coconut milk
- ½ teaspoon vanilla extract
- ¼ cup cherries, pitted and halved
- Cooking spray

Directions:
1. Put the milk in a pot, add the sugar and the coconut, stir and bring to a simmer over medium heat.
2. Add the rice and the other ingredients, simmer for 25 minutes stirring often, divide into bowls and serve.

Nutrition facts per serving: calories 505, fat 29.5, fiber 3.4, carbs 55.7, protein 6.6

Ginger and Almond Rice

Prep time: 10 minutes I **Cooking time:** 25 minutes I **Servings:** 4

Ingredients:
- 1 cup brown rice
- 2 cups almond milk
- 1 tablespoon ginger, grated
- 3 tablespoons coconut sugar
- 1 teaspoon cinnamon powder

Directions:
1. Put the milk in a pot, bring to a simmer over medium heat, add the rice and the other ingredients, stir, cook for 25 minutes, divide into bowls and serve.

Nutrition facts per serving: calories 449, fat 29, fiber 3.4, carbs 44.6, protein 6.2

Minced Hash Mix

Prep time: 10 minutes I **Cooking time:** 35 minutes I **Servings:** 4

Ingredients:
- 1 pound hash browns
- 4 eggs, whisked
- 1 red onion, chopped
- 1 chili pepper, chopped
- 1 tablespoon olive oil
- 6 ounces minced beef
- ¼ teaspoon chili powder
- A pinch of black pepper

Directions:
1. Heat up a pan with the oil over medium heat, add the onion and the minced beef, stir and brown for 5 minutes.
2. Add the hash browns and the other ingredients except the eggs and pepper, stir and cook for 5 minutes more.
3. Pour the eggs mixed with the black pepper over the minced mixture, introduce the pan in the oven and bake at 370 degrees F for 25 minutes.
4. Divide the mix between plates and serve the breakfast,

Nutrition facts per serving: calories 527, fat 31.3, fiber 3.8, carbs 51.2, protein 13.3

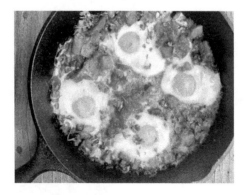

Mushroom and Cheddar Mix

Prep time: 10 minutes I **Cooking time:** 30 minutes I **Servings:** 4

Ingredients:
- 1 red onion, chopped
- 1 cup brown rice
- 2 garlic cloves, minced
- 2 tablespoons olive oil
- 2 cups chicken stock
- 1 tablespoon cilantro, chopped
- ½ cup cheddar cheese, grated
- ½ pound white mushroom, sliced
- Back pepper to the taste

Directions:
1. Heat up a pan with the oil over medium heat, add the onion, garlic and mushrooms, stir and cook for 5-6 minutes.
2. Add the rice and the rest of the ingredients, bring to a simmer and cook over medium heat for 25 minutes stirring often.
3. Divide the rice mix between bowls and serve for breakfast.

Nutrition facts per serving: calories 314, fat 12.2, fiber 1.8, carbs 42.1, protein 9.5

Tomato Eggs

Prep time: 10 minutes I **Cooking time:** 20 minutes I **Servings:** 4

Ingredients:
- ½ cup almond milk
- Black pepper to the taste
- 8 eggs, whisked
- 1 cup baby spinach, chopped
- 1 yellow onion, chopped
- 1 tablespoon olive oil
- 1 cup cherry tomatoes, cubed
- ¼ cup cheddar, grated

Directions:
1. Heat up a pan with the oil over medium heat, add the onion, stir and cook for 2-3 minutes.
2. Add the spinach and tomatoes, stir and cook for 2 minutes more.
3. Add the eggs mixed with the milk and black pepper and toss gently.
4. Sprinkle the cheddar on top, introduce the pan in the oven and cook at 390 degrees F for 15 minutes.
5. Divide between plates and serve.

Nutrition facts per serving: calories 195, fat 13, fiber 1.3, carbs 6.8, protein 13.7

Paprika Omelet

Prep time: 5 minutes I **Cooking time:** 15 minutes I **Servings:** 4

Ingredients:
- 4 eggs, whisked
- A pinch of black pepper
- 1 tablespoon olive oil
- 1 teaspoon sesame seeds
- 2 scallions, chopped
- 1 teaspoon sweet paprika
- 1 tablespoon cilantro, chopped

Directions:
1. Heat up a pan with the oil over medium heat, add the scallions, stir and sauté for 2 minutes.
2. Add the eggs mixed with the other ingredients, toss a bit, spread the omelet into the pan and cook for 7 minutes.
3. Flip, cook the omelet for 6 minutes more, divide between plates and serve.

Nutrition facts per serving: calories 101, fat 8.3, fiber 0.5, carbs 1.4, protein 5.9

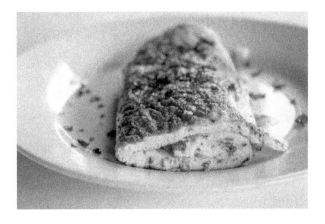

Cinnamon Zucchini and Oats

Prep time: 5 minutes I **Cooking time:** 20 minutes I **Servings:** 4

Ingredients:
- 1 cup steel cut oats
- 3 cups almond milk
- 1 tablespoon butter
- 2 teaspoons cinnamon powder
- 1 teaspoon pumpkin pie spice
- 1 cup zucchinis, grated

Directions:
1. Heat up a pan with the milk over medium heat, add the oats and the other ingredients, toss, bring to a simmer and cook for 20 minutes, stirring from time to time.
2. Divide the oatmeal into bowls and serve for breakfast.

Nutrition facts per serving: calories 508, fat 44.5, fiber 6.7, carbs 27.2, protein 7.5

Maple Almonds Bowl

Prep time: 5 minutes I **Cooking time:** 20 minutes I **Servings:** 4

Ingredients:
- 2 cups coconut milk
- 1 cup coconut, shredded
- ½ cup maple syrup
- 1 cup raisins
- 1 cup almonds
- ½ teaspoon vanilla extract

Directions:
1. Put the milk in a pot, bring to a simmer over medium heat, add the coconut and the other ingredients, and cook for 20 minutes, stirring from time to time.
2. Divide the mix into bowls and serve warm for breakfast.

Nutrition facts per serving: calories 697, fat 47.4, fiber 8.8, carbs 70, protein 9.6

Chickpeas and Cucumber Salad

Prep time: 5 minutes I **Cooking time:** 15 minutes I **Servings:** 4

Ingredients:
- 2 garlic cloves, minced
- 2 tomatoes, roughly cubed
- 1 cucumber, roughly cubed
- 2 shallots, chopped
- 2 cups chickpeas, cooked
- 1 tablespoon parsley, chopped
- 1/3 cup mint, chopped
- 1 avocado, pitted, peeled and diced
- 2 tablespoons olive oil
- Juice of 1 lime
- Black pepper to the taste

Directions:
1. Heat up a pan with the oil over medium heat, add the garlic and the shallots, stir and cook for 2 minutes.
2. Add the chickpeas and the other ingredients, toss, cook for 13 minutes more, divide into bowls and serve for breakfast.

Nutrition facts per serving: calories 561, fat 23.1, fiber 22.4, carbs 73.1, protein 21.8

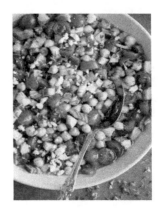

Millet Mix

Prep time: 10 minutes I **Cooking time:** 30 minutes I **Servings:** 4

Ingredients:
- 14 ounces coconut milk
- 1 cup millet
- 1 tablespoon cocoa powder
- ½ teaspoon vanilla extract

Directions:
1. Put the milk in a pot, bring to a simmer over medium heat, add the millet and the other ingredients, and cook for 30 minutes stirring often.
2. Divide into bowls and serve for breakfast.

Nutrition facts per serving: calories 422, fat 25.9, fiber 6.8, carbs 42.7, protein 8

Ginger Chia Pudding

Prep time: 15 minutes I **Cooking time:** 0 minutes I **Servings:** 4

Ingredients:
- 2 cups almond milk
- ½ cup chia seeds
- 2 tablespoons coconut sugar
- Zest of ½ lemon, grated
- 1 teaspoon vanilla extract
- ½ teaspoon ginger powder

Directions:
1. In a bowl, combine the chia seeds with the milk and the other ingredients, toss and leave aside for 15 minutes before serving.

Nutrition facts per serving: calories 366, fat 30.8, fiber 5.5, carbs 20.8, protein 4.6

Cinnamon Tapioca Bowls

Prep time: 2 hours I **Cooking time:** 0 minutes I **Servings:** 4

Ingredients:
- ½ cup tapioca pearls
- 2 cups coconut milk, hot
- 4 teaspoons coconut sugar
- ½ teaspoon cinnamon powder

Directions:
1. In a bowl, combine the tapioca with the hot milk and the other ingredients, stir and leave aside for 2 hours before serving.
2. Divide into small bowls and serve for breakfast.

Nutrition facts per serving: calories 439, fat 28.6, fiber 2.8, carbs 42.5, protein 3.8

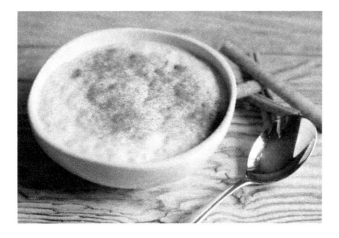

Coconut Hash

Prep time: 10 minutes I **Cooking time:** 25 minutes I **Servings:** 4

Ingredients:
- 1 pound hash browns
- 1 tablespoon avocado oil
- 1/3 cup coconut cream
- 1 yellow onion, chopped
- 1 cup cheddar cheese, grated
- Black pepper to the taste
- 4 eggs, whisked

Directions:
1. Heat up a pan with the oil over medium heat, add the hash browns and the onion, stir and sauté for 5 minutes.
2. Add the rest of the ingredients except the cheese, toss and cook for 5 minutes more.
3. Sprinkle the cheese on top, introduce the pan in the oven and cook at 390 degrees F for 15 minutes.
4. Divide the mix between plates and serve for breakfast.

Nutrition facts per serving: calories 539, fat 33.2, fiber 4.8, carbs 44.4, protein 16.8

Snow Peas and Scallions Bowls

Prep time: 10 minutes I **Cooking time:** 20 minutes I **Servings:** 4

Ingredients:
- 3 garlic cloves, minced
- 1 yellow onion, chopped
- 1 tablespoon olive oil
- 1 carrot, chopped
- 1 tablespoon balsamic vinegar
- 2 cups snow peas, halved
- ½ cup veggie stock
- 2 tablespoons scallions, chopped
- 1 tablespoon cilantro, chopped

Directions:
1. Heat up a pan with the oil over medium heat, add the onion and the garlic, stir and cook for 5 minutes.
2. Add the snow peas and the other ingredients, toss and cook over medium heat for 15 minutes.
3. Divide the mix into bowls and serve warm for breakfast.

Nutrition facts per serving: calories 89, fat 4.2, fiber 3.3, carbs 11.2, protein 3.3

Coconut Chickpeas Mix

Prep time: 10 minutes I **Cooking time:** 20 minutes I **Servings:** 6

Ingredients:
- 1 red onion, chopped
- 1 tablespoon olive oil
- 15 ounces chickpeas, cooked
- 14 ounces coconut milk
- ¼ cup quinoa
- 1 tablespoon ginger, grated
- 2 garlic cloves, minced
- 1 tablespoon turmeric powder
- 1 tablespoon cilantro, chopped

Directions:
1. Heat up a pan with the oil over medium heat, add the onion, stir and sauté for 5 minutes.
2. Add the chickpeas, quinoa and the other ingredients, stir, bring to a simmer and cook for 15 minutes.
3. Divide the mix into bowls and serve for breakfast.

Nutrition facts per serving: calories 472, fat 23, fiber 15.1, carbs 54.6, protein 16.6

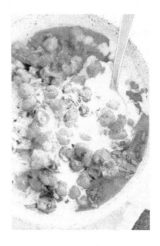

Lime Peppers Salad

Prep time: 5 minutes I **Cooking time:** 15 minutes I **Servings:** 4

Ingredients:
- 1 cup black olives, pitted and halved
- ½ cup green olives, pitted and halved
- 1 tablespoon olive oil
- 2 scallions, chopped
- 1 red bell pepper, cut into strips
- 1 green bell pepper, cut into strips
- Zest of 1 lime, grated
- Juice of 1 lime
- 1 bunch parsley, chopped
- 1 tomato, chopped

Directions:
1. Heat up a pan with the oil over medium heat, add the scallions, stir and sauté for 2 minutes.
2. Add the olives, peppers and the other ingredients, stir and cook for 13 minutes more.
3. Divide into bowls and serve for breakfast.

Nutrition facts per serving: calories 192, fat 6.7, fiber 3.3, carbs 9.3, protein 3.5

Green Beans Mix

Prep time: 10 minutes I **Cooking time:** 15 minutes I **Servings:** 4

Ingredients:
- 1 garlic clove, minced
- 1 red onion, chopped
- 1 tablespoon avocado oil
- 1 pound green beans, trimmed and halved
- 8 eggs, whisked
- 1 tablespoon cilantro, chopped
- A pinch of black pepper

Directions:
1. Heat up a pan with the oil over medium heat, add the onion and the garlic and sauté for 2 minutes.
2. Add the green beans and cook for 2 minutes more.
3. Add the eggs, black pepper and cilantro, toss, spread into the pan and cook for 10 minutes.
4. Divide the mix between plates and serve.

Nutrition facts per serving: calories 260, fat 12.1, fiber 4.7, carbs 19.4, protein 3.6

Eggs Salad

Prep time: 10 minutes I **Cooking time:** 0 minutes I **Servings:** 4

Ingredients:
- 2 carrots, cubed
- 2 green onions, chopped
- 1 bunch of parsley, chopped
- 2 tablespoons olive oil
- 4 eggs, hard boiled, peeled and cubed
- 1 tablespoon balsamic vinegar
- 1 tablespoon chives, chopped
- A pinch of black pepper

Directions:
1. In a bowl, combine the carrots with the eggs and the other ingredients, toss and serve for breakfast.

Nutrition facts per serving: calories 251, fat 9.6, fiber 4.1, carbs 15.2, protein 3.5

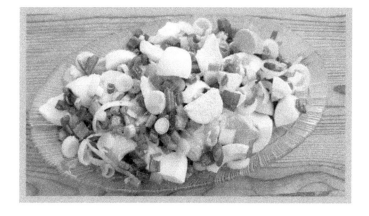

Vanilla Berries

Prep time: 5 minutes I **Cooking time:** 15 minutes I **Servings:** 4

Ingredients:
- 3 tablespoons coconut sugar
- 1 cup coconut cream
- 1 cup blueberries
- 1 cup blackberries
- 1 cup strawberries
- 1 teaspoon vanilla extract

Directions:
1. Put the cream in a pot, heat it up over medium heat, add the sugar and the other ingredients, toss, cook for 15 minutes, divide into bowls and serve for breakfast.

Nutrition facts per serving: calories 460, fat 16.7, fiber 6.5, carbs 40.3, protein 5.7

Apples and Blueberries Mix

Prep time: 5 minutes I **Cooking time:** 15 minutes I **Servings:** 4

Ingredients:
- 1 cup blueberries
- 1 teaspoon cinnamon powder
- 1 and ½ cups almond milk
- ¼ cup raisins
- 2 apples, cored, peeled and cubed
- 1 cup coconut cream

Directions:
1. Put the milk in a pot, bring to a simmer over medium heat, add the berries and the other ingredients, toss, cook for 15 minutes, divide into bowls and serve for breakfast.

Nutrition facts per serving: calories 482, fat 7.8, fiber 5.6, carbs 15.9, protein 4.9

Buckwheat Bowls

Prep time: 10 minutes I **Cooking time:** 25 minutes I **Servings:** 4

Ingredients:
- 1 cup buckwheat
- 3 cups coconut milk
- ½ teaspoon vanilla extract
- 1 tablespoon coconut sugar
- 1 teaspoon ginger powder
- 1 teaspoon cinnamon powder

Directions:
1. Put the milk and the sugar in a pot, bring to a simmer over medium heat, add the buckwheat and the other ingredients, cook for 25 minutes, stirring often, divide into bowls and serve for breakfast.

Nutrition facts per serving: calories 482, fat 14.9, fiber 4.5, carbs 56.3, protein 7.5

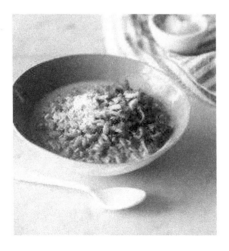

Cauliflower Salad

Prep time: 10 minutes I **Cooking time:** 20 minutes I **Servings:** 4

Ingredients:
- 1 pound cauliflower florets
- 1 tablespoon olive oil
- 2 spring onions, chopped
- 1 red bell pepper, sliced
- 1 yellow bell pepper, sliced
- 1 green bell pepper, sliced
- 1 tablespoon cilantro, chopped
- A pinch of black pepper

Directions:
1. Heat up a pan with the oil over medium heat, add the spring onions, stir and sauté for 2 minutes.
2. Add the cauliflower and the other ingredients, toss, cook for 16 minutes, divide into bowls and serve for breakfast.

Nutrition facts per serving: calories 271, fat 11.2 , fiber 3.4, carbs 11.5, protein 4

Chicken and Pepper Mix

Prep time: 10 minutes I **Cooking time:** 25 minutes I **Servings:** 4

Ingredients:
- 2 tablespoons olive oil
- 1 yellow onion, chopped
- 2 garlic cloves, minced
- 1 teaspoon Cajun seasoning
- 8 ounces chicken breast, skinless, boneless and ground
- ½ pound hash browns
- 2 tablespoons veggie stock
- 1 green bell pepper, chopped

Directions:
1. Heat up a pan with the oil over medium heat, add the onion, garlic and the meat and brown for 5 minutes.
2. Add the hash browns and the other ingredients, stir, and cook over medium heat for 20 minutes stirring often.
3. Divide between plates and serve for breakfast.

Nutrition facts per serving: calories 362, fat 14.3, fiber 6.3, carbs 25.6, protein 6.1

Beef Bowl

Prep time: 10 minutes I **Cooking time:** 20 minutes I **Servings:** 1

Ingredients:

- 4 ounces ground beef
- 1 onion, peeled and chopped
- 8 mushrooms, sliced
- Salt and ground black pepper, to taste
- 2 eggs, whisked
- 1 tablespoon coconut oil
- ½ teaspoon smoked paprika
- 1 avocado, pitted, peeled, and chopped
- 12 black olives, pitted and sliced

Directions:
1. Heat a pan with coconut oil over medium heat, add onions, mushrooms, salt, and pepper, stir, and cook for 5 minutes.
2. Add beef, and paprika, stir, cook for 10 minutes, transfer to a bowl. Heat up the pan again over medium heat, add eggs, some salt, pepper, and scramble.
3. Return beef mixture to pan and stir. Add avocado and olives, stir, and cook for 1 minute. Transfer to a bowl and serve.

Nutrition facts per serving: calories 1002, fat 74,9, fiber 19,4, carbs 36,9, protein 55,6

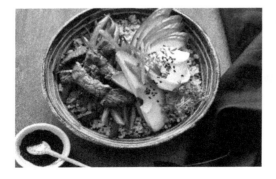

Smoked Salmon and Eggs Mix

Prep time: 10 minutes I **Cooking time:** 10 minutes I **Servings:** 3

Ingredients:

- 4 eggs, whisked
- ½ teaspoon avocado oil
- 4 ounces smoked salmon, chopped

For the sauce:

- 1 cup coconut milk
- ½ cup cashews, soaked and drained
- ¼ cup green onions, chopped
- 1 teaspoon garlic powder
- Salt and ground black pepper, to taste
- 1 tablespoon lemon juice

Directions:

1. In a blender, mix cashews with coconut milk, garlic powder, lemon juice and blend well.
2. Add salt, pepper, and green onions, blend again, transfer to a bowl, and place in refrigerator.
3. Heat up a pan with oil over medium–low heat, add eggs, whisk, and cook until they are almost done. Place under a preheated broiler, and cook until eggs are set.
4. Divide the eggs on plates, top with smoked salmon, and serve with the green onion sauce on top.

Nutrition facts per serving: calories 448, fat 37,3, fiber 2,7, carbs 13,1, protein 19,8

Cheesy Asparagus Mix

Prep time: 10 minutes I **Cooking time:** 25 minutes I **Servings:** 2

Ingredients:

- 12 asparagus spears
- 1 tablespoon olive oil
- 2 green onions, chopped
- 1 garlic clove, peeled and minced
- 6 eggs
- Salt and ground black pepper, to taste
- ½ cup feta cheese

Directions:
1. Heat a pan with some water over medium heat, add asparagus, cook for 8 minutes, drain well, chop 2 spears, and reserve the rest.
2. Heat a pan with oil over medium heat, add garlic, chopped asparagus, onions, stir, and cook for 5 minutes. Add eggs, salt, pepper, stir, cover, and cook for 5 minutes.
3. Arrange asparagus spears on top of the frittata, sprinkle cheese, place in oven at 350ºF, and bake for 9 minutes. Divide on plates and serve.

Nutrition facts per serving: calories 384, fat 28.3, fiber 3.4, carbs 9.7, protein 25.5

Stuffed Avocados

Prep time: 10 minutes I **Cooking time:** 20 minutes I **Servings:** 4

Ingredients:

- 2 avocados, cut in half and pitted
- 4 eggs
- Salt and ground black pepper, to taste
- 1 tablespoon fresh chives, chopped

Directions:
1. Scoop some flesh from the avocado halves and arrange in a baking dish.
2. Crack an egg in each avocado, season with salt, pepper, place in oven at 425ºF, and bake for 20 minutes. Sprinkle chives at end and serve.

Nutrition facts per serving: calories 268, fat 24, fiber 6.7, carbs 9, protein 7.5

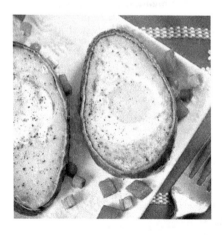

Eggs with Spinach and Chicken

Prep time: 10 minutes I **Cooking time:** 35 minutes I **Servings:** 6

Ingredients:

- 5 tablespoons butter
- 12 eggs
- Salt and ground black pepper, to taste
- 1 ounce spinach, torn
- 12 ham slices
- 10 oz chicken, chopped
- 1 onion, peeled and chopped
- 1 red bell pepper, seeded and chopped

Directions:
1. Heat a pan with 1 tablespoon butter over medium heat, add chicken, onion, stir, and cook for 5 minutes.
2. Add bell pepper, salt, pepper, stir, and cook for 3 minutes, transfer to a bowl. Melt rest of the butter, and divide into 12 cupcake molds.
3. Add a slice of ham to each cupcake mold, divide spinach in each and then add sausage mixture.
4. Crack an egg on top, place in an oven, and bake at 425 degrees Fahrenheit for 20 minutes. Let them cool briefly before serving.

Nutrition facts per serving: calories 378, fat 28,4, fiber 1,5, carbs 6,2, protein 24,5

Ham and Mushroom Scramble

Prep time: 10 minutes I **Cooking time:** 10 minutes I **Servings:** 1

Ingredients:

- 4 bell mushrooms, chopped
- 3 eggs, whisked
- Salt and ground black pepper, to taste
- 2 ham slices, chopped
- ¼ cup red bell pepper, seeded and chopped
- ½ cup spinach, chopped
- 1 tablespoon coconut oil

Directions:

1. Heat a pan with half of the oil over medium heat, add mushrooms, spinach, ham, bell pepper, stir, and cook for 4 minutes.
2. Heat another pan with the rest of the oil over medium heat, add eggs and scramble.
3. Add vegetables, ham, salt, and pepper, stir, cook for 1 minute, and serve.

Nutrition facts per serving: calories 430, fat 31,9, fiber 2,4, carbs 9, protein 29,5

Spinach and Chicken Frittata

Prep time: 10 minutes I **Cooking time:** 1 hour I **Servings:** 4

Ingredients:

- 9 ounces spinach
- 12 eggs
- 1 ounce chicken, boiled, chopped
- 1 teaspoon garlic, minced
- Salt and ground black pepper, to taste
- 5 ounces mozzarella cheese, shredded
- ½ cup Parmesan cheese, grated
- ½ cup ricotta cheese
- 4 tablespoons olive oil
- A pinch of nutmeg

Directions:
1. Squeeze liquid from spinach and put spinach in a bowl. In another bowl, mix eggs with salt, pepper, nutmeg, garlic, and whisk.
2. Add spinach, Parmesan cheese, ricotta cheese, and whisk.
3. Pour mixture into a pan, sprinkle with mozzarella cheese and chicken on top, place in oven, and bake at 375ºF for 45 minutes.
4. Let frittata cool down for a few minutes before serving.

Nutrition facts per serving: calories 525, fat 40,7, fiber 1,4, carbs 6,7, protein 35,9

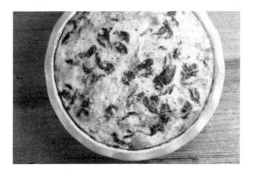

Boiled Eggs

Prep time: 10 minutes I **Cooking time:** 4 minutes I **Servings:** 12

Ingredients:

- 4 tea bags
- 4 tablespoons salt
- 12 eggs
- 2 tablespoons ground cinnamon
- 6 star anise
- 1 teaspoon ground black pepper
- 1 tablespoon peppercorns
- 8 cups water
- 1 cup tamari sauce

Directions:

1. Put water in a pot, add eggs, bring to a boil over medium heat, and cook until hard boiled.
2. Allow to cool and crack them without peeling. In a large pot, mix water with tea bags, salt, pepper, peppercorns, cinnamon, star anise, and tamari sauce.
3. Add cracked eggs, cover pot, bring to a simmer over low heat, and cook for 30 minutes. Discard tea bags and cook eggs for 3 hours and 30 minutes.
4. Let the eggs cool, peel, and serve.

Nutrition facts per serving: calories 122, fat 4.6, fiber 0.8, carbs 6.7, protein 13.9

Shrimp and Mushroom Mix

Prep time: 10 minutes I **Cooking time:** 15 minutes I **Servings:** 4

Ingredients:

- 1 cup mushrooms, sliced
- 4 bacon slices, chopped
- 4 ounces smoked salmon, chopped
- 4 ounces shrimp, deveined
- Salt and ground black pepper, to taste
- ½ cup coconut cream

Directions:
1. Heat a pan over medium heat, add bacon, stir, and cook for 5 minutes.
2. Add mushrooms, stir, and cook for 5 minutes. Add salmon, stir, and cook for 3 minutes.
3. Add shrimp and cook for 2 minutes.
4. Add salt, pepper, and coconut cream, stir, cook for 1 minute, take off heat, and divide on plates.

Nutrition facts per serving: Calories – 242, Fat – 16.8, Fiber – 0.8, Carbs – 2.9, Protein – 19.9

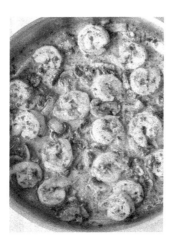

Chorizo and Pork Mix

Prep time: 10 minutes I **Cooking time:** 30 minutes I **Servings:** 8

Ingredients:

- ½ cup tomato paste
- ½ tsp garlic powder
- 1 tsp dried basil
- 1 tsp dried oregano
- 1 tsp cumin
- 2 tsp chili powder
- 1 pound ground pork
- 1 pound chorizo, chopped
- Salt and ground black pepper, to taste
- 8 eggs
- 1 tomato, cored and chopped
- 3 tablespoons butter
- ½ cup onion, chopped
- 1 avocado, pitted, peeled, and chopped

Directions:

1. In a bowl, mix spices and tomato paste to make enchilada sauce. In a second bowl, mix pork with chorizo, stir, and spread on a lined baking sheet.
2. Spread enchilada sauce on top, place in oven at 350ºF, and bake for 20 minutes.
3. Heat a pan with butter over medium heat, add eggs, and scramble them.
4. Take pork mixture out of oven and spread scrambled eggs over them.
5. Sprinkle salt, pepper, tomato, onion, and avocado on top, divide on plates, and serve.

Nutrition facts per serving: calories 513, fat 37.6, fiber 2.8, carbs 8.4, protein 35.6

Sausage and Spinach Mix

Prep time: 10 minutes I **Cooking time:** 40 minutes I **Servings:** 4

Ingredients:

- 10 eggs
- 1 pound pork sausage, chopped, hand-made
- 1 onion, peeled and chopped
- 3 cups spinach, torn
- Salt and ground black pepper, to taste
- 3 tablespoons avocado oil

Directions:
1. Heat a pan with 1 tablespoon oil over medium heat, add sausage, stir, and brown it for 4 minutes.
2. Add onion, stir, and cook for 3 minutes. Add spinach, stir, and cook for 1 minute.
3. Grease a baking dish with the rest of the oil, and spread the sausage mixture in it.
4. Whisk eggs and add them to sausage mixture.
5. Stir gently, place in oven at 350ºF, and bake for 30 minutes. Let the casserole cool for a few minutes before serving.

Nutrition facts per serving: calories 572, fat 44.5, fiber 1.6, carbs 4.8, protein 36.9

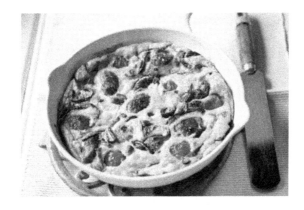

CPSIA information can be obtained
at www.ICGtesting.com
Printed in the USA
BVHW040948150121
597946BV00004B/25